WHAT'S THERE TO EAT AGAIN? Practical Steps To Losing Belly Fat Within 21 Days

LILIAN WEALTH

Table of Contents

Chapter 1

Where Does Belly Fat Originate From?

Belly fat is an issue, and not only because of how it looks. There are various reasons why individuals accumulate belly fat, including poor nutrition, lack of exercise, and stress. Belly fat refers to fat around the abdomen.

There are two forms of abdominal fat:

1. Visceral: This fat surrounds a person's organs. It surrounds your organs and elevates your risk for heart disease, type 2 diabetes, and several malignancies.

2. Subcutaneous: This is fat that resides beneath the skin.

Health issues from visceral fat are more hazardous than having subcutaneous fat.

Improving diet, boosting exercise, and making other lifestyle adjustments may all assist.

Reasons Why Belly Fat Develops

1. You're Eating Too Much

If you take in more calories than you burn off, you put on pounds everywhere — especially in your stomach. You need to decrease roughly 500 calories a day to lose a pound. That may seem like a lot but look at removing the highest-calorie foods from your diet first. Cookies, french fries, soda, and juice contain numerous calories in a few sips or nibbles. Sugary food such as cakes and candies, and beverages such as soda and fruit juice, can:

- increase weight gain

- slow a person's metabolism

- reduce a person's capacity to burn fat

Low-protein, high-carb diets may also affect weight. Protein helps a person feel satiated for longer, and those who do not consume lean protein in their diet may eat more food overall. Replace them initially with low-calorie, nutrient-dense meals like broccoli, apples, brown rice, and brothy soups.

2. You've Had a Few More Birthdays

Age may provide knowledge, but it isn't nice to your midline. With each passing year, your muscle mass reduces and your metabolism slows, so you don't burn as many calories as you used to. That means you may eat the same amount and yet watch the number on the scale creep higher. Age-acquired weight tends to gather around the midsection. To avoid undesired growth, cut down on calories or add extra muscle-building activity.

3. Blame Your Genes

If you eat correctly and exercise and those obstinate pounds still won't budge, your genes might be at fault. There is some evidence that a person's genes may play an influence on whether they become fat. Scientists suspect genes may impact behavior, metabolism, and the likelihood of acquiring obesity-related disorders.

Another indicator is if other family members battle with their weight. Genes determine how your body burns calories, how fast you feel full, and whether you acquire weight in your thighs, butt, or tummy. Even though belly obesity runs in your family, you may overcome your genes with the appropriate diet and enough exercise.

Environmental factors and behavior also have a role in the chances of persons becoming fat.

4. You've Started 'The Change'

In women, the combination of aging and the loss of estrogen during menopause adds up to a weight increase. Genes, loss of muscle mass, and overeating can contribute to weight creep in your 40s and 50s. The excess pounds that would have rested in your hips earlier in life now cluster around your midsection, also attributable to hormone changes. That weight shift does more than make your jeans tighter. It may also enhance your risk for heart disease.

5. You Don't Move Enough

Americans spend more than 10 hours a day in a sitting posture. Although eating plays a key factor in weight growth, lack of mobility contributes, too. If a person eats more calories than they burn off, they will put on weight.

A sedentary lifestyle makes it hard for a person to get rid of extra fat, especially around the belly. To prevent putting on additional pounds in your belly and elsewhere in your body, obtain at least 150 minutes of moderate-intensity or 75 minutes of high-intensity cardiovascular activity per week.

6. Sleep Is Hard to Come By

Too little shut-eye might be part of the reason you've gained weight. Your body generates hormones that help you feel full. Lack of rest might make them less effective. That's why, when you're sleep-deprived, you may overeat and gain weight, particularly in your belly. When you don't get enough sleep, you may also crave more high-calorie comfort foods. The short duration of sleep is linked to an increase in food intake, which may play a part in the development of abdominal fat. Not getting enough good sleep also may, potentially, lead to unhealthy eating behaviors, such as emotional eating.

7. You're Stress Eating

Too much stress isn't good for your mental state or your weight. Stress triggers the release of cortisol, a hormone that makes you crave high-fat, carb-heavy foods like pizza, fries, and cookies. People frequently look for food for consolation when they feel worried. Cortisol causes those surplus calories to linger around the abdomen and other parts of the body for later utilization.

Another way stress contributes to weight gain is by keeping you awake at night. People who sleep fewer hours are likely to have higher abdominal fat.

8. You Haven't Kicked the Habit

Some individuals who smoke are hesitant to stop because they fear that they'll gain weight. But even while smokers have a lower body mass index than nonsmokers, their stomachs are larger. Smokers accumulate more visceral fat, the sort that's related to heart disease and other chronic health concerns, than nonsmokers. So, in case you needed another reason to resign, now you've got one.

9. You Eat Too Many Trans Fats

These artificial fats elevate bad (LDL) cholesterol and enhance your risk for heart disease and type 2 diabetes. Foods fried with trans fats are rich in fat and calories and may induce weight gain. Trans fats, in particular, may promote inflammation and may contribute to obesity. Trans fats are found in numerous meals, including fast food and baked products like muffins and crackers.

The FDA has banned added trans fats in foods, but some products made before the ban could still be on store shelves. Read food labels. Reading food labels can help a person determine whether the ingredients list includes partially hydrogenated vegetable oil, and that food contains trans fat. Try to choose a different item. The American Heart Association suggests that consumers replace trans fats with nutritious whole-grain meals, monounsaturated fats, and polyunsaturated fats.

10. Your Gut Bacteria Aren't Helpful

Your intestines are home to billions of germs. Some of these microorganisms live in peace with you and help your body digest meals. Others break down food so much that your body absorbs more calories from it and stores more energy in the form of fat. There's evidence that probiotics, present in fermented foods like kimchi and yogurt, could get rid of abdominal fat. These friendly bacteria won't replace calorie restrictions, but they could help.

11.   It's Your Medicine

The solution to your weight gain might be buried within your medication cabinet. Certain medicines are known for inducing weight gain. These include certain diabetic treatments, some antidepressants, steroids, and epilepsy meds. A few drugs deposit fat straight to the abdominal region, including beta-blockers, which treat high blood pressure.

Chapter 2

Benefits of a Flat Stomach

Maintaining a trim midsection does more than make you look great—it might help you live longer. Larger waistlines are related to an increased risk of heart disease, diabetes, and even cancer. Losing weight, particularly belly fat, significantly improves blood vessel activity and also improves sleep quality.

Losing abdominal fat is more than simply looking better; it's about improving your health and quality of life. The two primary advantages you'll get with a reduced quantity of belly fat are the reversal of metabolic syndrome and the preservation of your heart.

It's hard to target abdominal fat particularly when you diet. But decreasing weight overall can help lower your waistline; more critically, it will help reduce the harmful layer of visceral fat, a form of fat inside the abdominal cavity that you can't see but that heightens health risks

Here are the advantages your body may anticipate seeing:

1. You'll have improved blood sugar management

More than one in three Americans have prediabetes when blood sugar is not quite high enough to be termed diabetes but high enough to be concerning—and 90 percent don't realize they have it. One of the major risk factors, however, is being overweight.

Excess belly fat raises insulin resistance, and because insulin is the key that unlocks cells to let sugar in, the more resistant you get to insulin, the more sugar builds up in the bloodstream. As you reduce visceral fat, insulin resistance diminishes, enabling sugar to enter cells more readily and allowing blood glucose levels to stay in a safe range. Dropping merely five percent of your body weight will do.

2. You'll reduce your chance of diabetes

Dropping your blood sugar also lessens your chance of acquiring full-blown diabetes, which has been demonstrated in studies to be related to abdominal obesity. This fat buildup disrupts insulin signaling, lowers glucose absorption by muscle cells, and hinders the liver's capacity to determine when it should stop releasing further glucose into the circulation. Each of these may contribute to a higher risk for diabetes.

In addition, decreasing weight also enhances the function of beta cells, which are the cells in the pancreas that create insulin. Here are other health secrets your pancreas wishes it could tell you.

3. Your liver will be healthier

Fat around the abdomen affects the way the liver, your natural "detox" mechanism, operates. Visceral fat affects the body via lipotoxicity. In this mechanism, metabolic byproducts from visceral fat cells are delivered straight into circulation.

The liver and other organs are not meant to collect substantial quantities of free fatty acids. Too much buildup of fatty acids in the liver might induce nonalcoholic fatty liver disease. In extreme situations, inflammation from the fatty liver might develop into cirrhosis or scarring of the liver. Maintaining a healthy weight is one of the greatest methods to avoid liver disease.

4. You'll lessen your blood pressure and heart disease risk

Researchers have discovered that even a five percent weight reduction decreases your risk for cardiovascular disease and improves general metabolic function—and other researchers point to abdominal fat as a specific problem when it comes to your risk.

Losing weight may help reduce your blood pressure. Too much adipose tissue puts additional stress on the heart as it attempts to pump a bigger volume of blood to our tissues and organs. Even a modest five percent weight reduction may help manage or prevent cardiovascular disease in overweight and obese persons by lowering these risk factors.

In addition, extra belly fat may elevate inflammatory hormones in the body and raise the level of cholesterol, triglycerides, and homocysteine—an independent risk factor for heart disease.

5. You'll increase your sleep quality

You may not imagine that your jeans size influences how easily you sleep off at night. But research from Johns Hopkins indicated that decreasing abdominal fat improved sleep quality, evaluated by levels of daily weariness, insomnia, restless sleep, and other characteristics. Obesity and being overweight are also connected with the dangerous disorder sleep apnea, in which soft tissues of the neck shut, impeding breathing.

Losing weight may help minimize snoring and sleep apnea, and can enhance the quality of your sleep in general. Here are minor sleep apnea warning symptoms you might be missing.

6. You'll have a lower cancer risk

Having a lot of belly fat, independent of total weight, is connected with colon and rectal cancer, and possibly with others such as pancreatic and breast cancer as well, according to the American Cancer Society.

Although the specific mechanisms are unclear, it is hypothesized that the enhanced inflammation and increased hormone synthesis brought about by extra belly fat may raise the risk for some malignancies. Losing even a tiny amount of weight may help.

7. You'll be less likely to get arthritis

Not surprisingly, carrying around a heavy belly can put a lot of strain on your joints (just ask anyone pregnant!). Excessive weight may be a load on your joints, which can subsequently lead to arthritis. Losing 10 pounds lessens the strain on your knees by 40 pounds. Plus, visceral fat may promote persistent inflammation, which might make arthritis worse. The inflammatory chemicals generated by adipose tissue may impact arthritis development. Fewer pro-inflammatory markers are generated following weight reduction, which may lower the risk for arthritis.

8. You'll have improved sexual health

The hormone disturbances induced by visceral fat may explain why women who are overweight or obese may have irregular periods. Being obese may induce atypical menstrual periods from the presence of extra fat that generates significant levels of estrogen, producing hormone.

This may have a factor in fertility for people attempting to conceive. The hormones that govern our diet [such as insulin] are tied to our sex hormones. While weight may only be a contribution to infertility, it's something most women can modify with diet and exercise.

Men aren't off the hook, either. For males, [being overweight] might lead to erectile dysfunction and diminished reproductive capacity.

9. You'll be in a better mood

Although it's a bit of a chicken-or-egg scenario, research has found that losing a bit of weight does improve mood and reduce depressive symptoms. This may be due to the weight loss itself or the change in lifestyle factors that led to it, such as stress reduction and exercise. Exercising releases endorphins, which help keep depression at bay. Beyond physical activity, looking good can also help your self-esteem. The regulation of hormones and improved sleep can also contribute to the better sense of well-being that comes with dropping belly fat.

Chapter 3

Myths About a Flat Belly

If conquering belly fat were simple, we'd all look like magazine cover models. But it doesn't imply flat abs are out of reach; it just takes a complete assault strategy.

A protruding belly is a typical source of worry for most individuals. So, anytime they come across some diet or exercise craze that promises immediate results, most people fall for it. Tall promises like 'develop washboard abs' in a month or reduce abdominal fat in a week may appear enticing. But what you need to realize is that these false promises barely produce any results. There are many myths and misunderstandings concerning weight reduction and it is nearly hard to resist falling for them. Here in this chapter, I have attempted to dispel several prevalent beliefs connected to belly fat.

Myth 1: Target weight loss is not attainable.

Truth: No activity can assist you to reduce down inches for any particular location. You will lose weight steadily from every part of your body- thighs, arms, belly. Target weight reduction is not achievable. Exercises like crunches and v-ups certainly exercise the muscle around the abdomen, but it does not imply you will drop kilograms quicker.

Myth 2: Belly fat is exactly like other fat in the body fat

Truth: It is typical to imagine that all forms of fats contained in the body are the same, yet they are not. The fat collected around the abdominal region is significantly more harmful than the one found in other sections of the body. Belly fat, also known as visceral fat, is collected deep beneath the skin, and around the organs and commonly leads to health difficulties including insulin resistance, type 2 diabetes, and cardiovascular problems.

Myth 3: Certain cuisine will melt abdominal fat

Truth: Some individuals claim that consuming foods like capsicum and cayenne pepper will assist you to burn abdominal fat quicker. However, these are mere claims and do not show any result. There is just a slim possibility that it can offer a boost to your metabolism, which might quicken the weight reduction process. But won't assist you to reduce weight, particularly in the abdominal region.

Myth 4: Wearing a waist trainer may be effective

Truth: You can come across dozens of waist trainer adverts on television, promising instant results. Let us notify you that these beautiful pieces of equipment do not truly operate. There is no shortcut to reducing belly fat, at least not by using waist trainers. For dropping kilograms, exercise and diet are needed.

Myth 5: Avoiding fatty meals may help decrease tummy fat

Truth: Eating fatty meals is not something that leads to a protruding belly in the first place. It is a consequence of your bad food, inactivity, sleeping pattern, and other lifestyle behaviors. Only by making modifications in every area and practicing good living habits, you will be able to reduce some inches from your waistline.

Myth 6: Nuts Are Fattening

Truth: Nuts have earned a poor reputation for their overall fat content, but nutrition research reveals that the quality—not quantity—of fat is what is most crucial to human health. The FDA just declared they are re-evaluating the word 'healthy' as it refers to foods containing good-for-you fats, like pistachios. What's more, foods like in-shell pistachios may help you mislead yourself into feeling full since the residual shells may give a visual indication for quantities, perhaps helping to decrease consumption.

Myth 7: Drinking Beer Causes A Beer Belly

Truth: While beer drinking doesn't seem to assist in decreasing your waist, a beer belly isn't always caused by beer; it's more likely caused by ingesting too many empty calories. Although, if you prefer guzzling six-packs daily, then you need to reassess your beer drinking habits. Do you know what has been proven to promote a bulging gut? Soda. It's termed "soda belly".

Myth 8: Avoiding Fatty Foods Will Result in Losing Belly Fat

Truth: Consuming a decent quantity of healthy fats is crucial to weight reduction. Healthy fats like olive oil and avocado oil enhance lifespan, bright skin, hair, and nails, and fight against cardiovascular disease and diabetes by keeping your blood glucose levels steady. They make you feel full and demand more energy from your body to metabolize. The goal is to integrate precisely the proper quantity into the diet. One serving of fat equals one tablespoon of olive oil, 10 olives, or 1/4 avocado. Most individuals should aim for two to three servings a day.

Myth 9: Ab Exercises Are All You Need for Abs

Truth: No number of crunches can give you abs if you have layers of fat covering your abdomen. For your abs to appear, you must concentrate on your nutrition first. Everyone is born with abdominal muscles that differ in form and appearance, and training will only aid to grow the muscle itself. Eating a clean, balanced diet can aid in fat reduction around the abdominal muscles and enable them to shine through.

Myth 10: Some People Are Born to Have Belly Fat

Truth: The sites where your body likes to store fat are set by your genes, but it does not indicate that you will be overweight in those areas. For example, someone who is apple-shaped tends to retain more fat in the abdomen area, but if they follow the right diet and exercise plan, they may avoid weight gain.

Myth 11: Seed Oils Are Always Healthy

Truth: The term "seed" might make something seem instantly healthful, but that's not the case when it comes to some oils. Processed and industrial seed oil like maize, cottonseed, soybean oil, and peanut oil might severely influence our ratio of omega-3 to omega-6 fats. This may lead to persistent inflammation, which is a factor in resistive weight loss, and they can include GMOs that disrupt the gut microbiota. Opt for healthy oils like flaxseed oil, olive oil, avocado oil, and hemp seed oil.

Myth 12: Low-Fat Packaged Products Are Good For You

Truth: You truly need to consume some fat.

Fat causes the sense of fullness to keep you from overeating, stabilizes blood sugar—preventing fat-storing insulin to spike—and helps you to absorb vital fat-soluble nutrients including vitamins A, D, E, and K. It's also crucial to understand that when food makers take away fat, they need to compensate for a loss in taste. They typically do so by putting in enormous quantities of salt, sugar, or both.

Myth 13: Low-Fat or Nonfat Dairy Is Good For You

Truth: Some professionals counsel their clients to stay away from low or nonfat dairy products. Unless your milk is organic and comes from pasture-raised/grass-fed cows, [producers] will likely be feeding synthetic growth hormones, steroids, antibiotics, and genetically engineered maize to those animals to substantially accelerate their weight gain. Also, when it's pasteurized, you lose many beneficial nutrients and enzymes that help with digestion.

Myth 14: Caffeine Boosts Weight Loss

Truth: There are a solid 35 Things You Don't Know About Caffeine and one is probably how caffeine can confuse your cortisol production. (Cortisol, FYI, tells your body to hang onto fat.) In moderation, caffeine can be a great thing. Not only can caffeine give you an energy boost, but it has also been shown to help with sports performance. That said, it can also have the opposite effect and end up wearing you out. This is especially true if you are already worn down and under stress; it can perpetuate an imbalance of hormones, namely cortisol, that contribute to fat storage, especially around the middle.

Myth 15: A Juice Cleanse Is the Ultimate Way to Lose Weight

Truth: The difficulty with juices and smoothies is that it's possible to drink quite significant quantities of sugar and calories without realizing it. As if the calorie and sugar counts aren't enough to cause you to forgo the juice cleanse, many juices don't include the fiber that makes fresh fruit so beneficial for you. After all, fiber helps keep you full for longer periods and mitigates blood-sugar increases. A juice may include more than one serving of fruit, which adds up to a lot of sugar. But without any fiber, you won't feel full or get the advantages of balancing your blood glucose levels and shedding weight.

Myth 16: 8 Hours of Sleep Will Cause You to Lose Weight

Truth: Sleep is better than no sleep, but studies suggest that the quality of sleep you receive is incredibly essential, too. Whether you have sleep apnea—meaning you're never actually getting a restorative sleep—or just can't turn off your thoughts at night, it's not enough to merely remain in your bed for eight hours. Sleeping properly during the night, without a restless mind or sporadically waking up, is vital to making sure you wake up refreshed and less worried. Drinking alcohol before bedtime can make it simpler for you to fall asleep, but increase the number of nightly arousals.

Myth 17: Drinking Green Tea Melts Fat

Truth: Green tea is great but it's not a magic potion; you still have to alter other parts of your diet and life.

Drinking green tea is terrific, particularly if it's instead of juices and sodas, but although studies have shown that drinking approximately three cups of it a day may help raise your metabolism, it's not enough to melt off belly fat. People must be aware that drinking green tea is only truly effective if it's consumed as a supplement to a healthy diet and exercise plan.

Myth 18: The Time You Eat Can Have A Huge Impact

Truth: Food is food whether you have it at 1 a.m. or 1 p.m. More important than the time of day is the quality and quantity of the food you consume. Listen to your body. The total number of calories matters and most people tend to continuously snack throughout the night as their inhibitions go down. But if you need to stay up late and work on a deadline and are truly hungry, then you should eat; just make sure you're not eating out of boredom or because you're thirsty. A decent guideline is to ask yourself whether you'd eat an apple. If you wouldn't eat an apple, the likelihood is you're simply feeling a yearning and aren't genuinely hungry.

Myth 19: Eating A Vegan Diet Blasts Belly Fat

Truth: Although studies have preferred certain diets over others, there is no one specific diet that can automatically help you blast away belly fat. The most essential thing is to concentrate on eating enough fresh vegetables, lean protein, and healthy fats, and reducing the quantities of processed carbs and saturated fats you're ingesting.

Myth 20: Small Meals Are The Answer

Truth: We typically hear that eating more frequent, smaller meals would melt off belly fat, but that's not always true.

You don't need to eat little meals every two hours. You may more efficiently enhance your metabolism by eating three balanced meals and one snack every day. Not only will you feel more content and fuller longer by having a complete meal, but you'll still be keeping your blood sugar levels consistent and won't risk overeating to the same degree as you may if you graze on foods throughout the day.

Myth 21: You Need To Eat Less

Truth: If you severely cut down on the number of calories—instead of enhancing the quality of your calories—you'll likely cause harm to your metabolism and lose out on long-term success. Yes, calorie tracking may be one technique to reduce weight. But scientists regularly warn that your body will go into famine mode and slow down metabolism to cling onto the calories it receives when it eventually gets them. Not eating enough is damaging to your metabolism. It might slow it down, making it harder for you to lose weight and keep it. Keep your metabolism up by eating balanced and thoroughly thought-out meals that emphasize high-quality, fresh foods.

Myth 22: Eating Cherries Reduces Belly Fat

Truth: There are some fantastic fat-burning meals, but no cure-alls. There are always trends that lend some trendy foods supposedly mystical qualities. And as of late, you might have read splashy headlines touting the benefits of tart cherries. Unfortunately, eating tart cherries alone will not help you lose fat around the belly. You need to consume an overall healthy diet that is within your calorie range. Tart cherries are excellent for you in other ways, much like other fruits; they are rich in fiber, vitamins, and antioxidants, meaning they're a terrific addition to your diet (instead of sugar, for example) (instead of candy, for example).

Myth 23: Shots Of Apple Cider Vinegar Melt Fat

Truth: Drinking apple cider vinegar alone will not burn away abdominal fat. Some studies have suggested that vinegar, in general, may assist increase insulin sensitivity. But it is ideal to couple this plan with a good diet and exercise to obtain optimum effects.

Myth 24: You Have Bad Genes So All Is Lost

Truth: Genes have a role in your form, but using your genes as a blanket explanation for your shape isn't doing you any favors. When your gut bacteria (aka microbiome) is out of balance with more bad bacteria than good (aka dysbiosis), fat storage is promoted. This dysbiosis can be from many factors including lack of sleep, not enough exercise, or too much stress, but a diet high in processed foods, refined sugar, and foods you don't tolerate are the most influential factors. Recent research has shown that those with more diversity of microbes in their gut microbiome, had lower visceral fat (the fat around your organs in your abdominal area that is associated with metabolic disease) (the fat around your organs in your abdominal area that is associated with metabolic disease). While you can't alter your genes, your microbiota composition is quite flexible. Improve your gut health and obtain your carbohydrates from veggies, consume fermented foods, get some probiotics in your life, and attempt an elimination diet to help identify your food sensitivities.

Myth 25: Fruits Can Emulsify Belly Fat

Truth: While citric acid is a naturally occurring acid in fruits and vegetables, it doesn't emulsify stored fat. A common myth is that citric acid in fruits like cranberries emulsifies your belly fat. The fact is that it's engaged in the TCA cycle, which provides energy via the oxidation of carbs, lipids, and proteins. This also implies that any lotion that professes to blast abdominal fat or to burn away cellulite with acid-rich cranberries won't truly deliver. That said, while citric acid-rich fruits won't blast fat on their own, eat them instead of processed sweets and salty snacks and you're bound to see some results.

Myth 26: Cinnamon Burns Calories

Truth: Cinnamon helps blood sugar control but is not connected to calorie burning.

Cinnamon and herbs and spices, in general, are a great way to add flavor to your foods without packing on calories; that doesn't mean they're a cure-all. It's a common myth that consuming a teaspoon of ground cinnamon every day helps you lose fat quickly. The truth is that while studies show that cinnamon may play a role in blood sugar control, cinnamon is not connected to greater calorie burn. Additionally, you would need to take a lot more than just a teaspoon of cinnamon to achieve the minor advantages.

Myth 27: Going Gluten-Free Helps Blast Belly Fat

Truth: Oftentimes, the weight reduction observed by persons avoiding gluten comes from the overall drop in calories from avoiding all carbs in general. The food business relies on the fact that many consumers wrongly feel that 'gluten-free' is code for healthy, so they disguise highly processed goods as good-for-you snacks. It's fairly usual for individuals who start on gluten-free diets to acquire belly fat since they're substituting whole grain, gluten-containing complex carbs with processed, refined gluten-free items.

Myth 28: Lemon Water Melts Fat

Truth: It's probably simply that you're drinking water in the first place. It would be hard to tally the number of individuals who swear by beginning their day with hot water and lemon. And although it's undoubtedly a healthy way to start the morning, there's a dearth of scientific proof that supports any claims that it burns away fat. The typical American does not drink enough water in general. Therefore, drinking a glass of lemon water in the morning on an empty stomach may just help in hydration and suppressing appetite, leading to overall less calorie consumption.

Myth 29: Dark Fruits Burn More Belly Fat

Truth: No data says darker fruits burn more fat. All fruit includes phytonutrients, so it's crucial to consume a range of hues to ensure you're receiving as many nutrients as possible. There isn't research demonstrating that darker fruits burn fat. Rather, consider consuming berries that are strong in fiber for a delicious and slow-digesting choice.

Myth 30: Belly Fat Doesn't Matter If Your BMI Is Normal

Truth: BMI is important in helping someone comprehend that they are overweight or obese, but that's about all it's good for. It's not an accurate approach to assessing overall health. We may believe that fat is fat, but its location of it also has health ramifications. Although BMI is a reasonable indicator of overweight or obesity status, having fat in the belly area is more hazardous to your health than being slightly overweight without significant belly fat. Even if your BMI is normal, central obesity can be a risk factor for metabolic syndrome, diabetes, and cardiovascular disease.

Myth 31: Calories Are Calories

Truth: 100 calories from two manufactured, preservative-packed cookies are not comparable to 100 calories from an apple. Who do you believe is healthier: someone who eats 1,200 calories worth of candy and chocolates or someone who eats 2,000 calories worth of veggies and lean protein? It's not only about the number of calories, but also about the quality of those calories. Although keeping your calories in control is crucial for general weight reduction, nutritious food sources are key to decreasing belly fat and developing lean muscle development. Studies reveal that if you compare two persons who eat the same number of calories worth of saturated fat and unsaturated good fats, the one who consumes more saturated fat would have more belly fat.

Chapter 4

Flat Stomach Natural Remedies

Living with fat around your stomach might be a risk factor for various chronic ailments, including cancer and heart problems. However, if you're living with extra abdominal fat and have been seeking strategies to shed it, you undoubtedly understand it's not always as straightforward as some weight loss experts would have you think.

For one, the size (or "flatness") of your stomach may depend on several different circumstances, including the time of day, whether you've exercised lately, and what meals or beverages you've ingested throughout the day Furthermore, several previous research have indicated that spot reduction — or focused fat loss in a particular location of the body — is not viable. This is because fat cells are stored throughout the body and may be broken down and utilized as energy during exercise from any portion of the body, not just the place where you're exercising.

Various ways may boost weight reduction and stimulate muscle gain. When paired with a balanced diet and health-promoting lifestyle, this might help lower belly fat while improving overall health. Here are some science-backed strategies to help you shed excess belly fat.

- **Include aerobic workouts in your everyday routine**

If you want to burn fat rapidly there is no getting around an aerobic workout. Studies suggest that this is the most effective kind of exercise to decrease abdominal fat. By burning numerous calories your overall health will improve. Hence, start practicing high-intensity exercises like jogging, swimming, or aerobic courses, but bear in mind that frequency and length are vital for fulfilling outcomes.

- **Start the day with a high-protein breakfast**

Start your day with some Greek yogurt, protein smoothies, scrambled egg whites, or oatmeal. After consuming proteins in the morning, you will feel full till lunch without any hunger sensations. Proteins enhance your metabolic rate while keeping muscle mass during weight reduction. You may also include proteins such as eggs, fish, poultry, legumes, or dairy with every other meal.

- **Drink enough water**

Even if you don't intend to lose weight, being hydrated is vital for your overall health. Drinking 4 to 5 liters of water each day is advised and will burn more calories.

Also, drinking shortly before eating lessens your hunger as well as calorie consumption. Make careful to avoid any other drinks having plenty of sweets and calories. Drinking warm water with lemon in the morning on an empty stomach helps jumpstart your metabolism and digestive system as well.

- **Reduce your salt consumption**

Consumed salt holds water and makes your gut feels bloated. Before making a purchase always make sure the nutrition label does not specify excessive sodium levels as processed food comprises a salt, added sugar, and bad fats.

- **Consume soluble fiber**

Similar to proteins, soluble fibers help you feel full for a few hours so that you don't have to ingest needless additional calories in your meal. Soluble fibers absorb water and

produce a gel that inhibits fat absorption —
a positive thing for someone attempting to
lose weight. You may find them in barley,
almonds, seeds, beans, and lentils.

- **Cut calories, but not too much**

Typically, if you're aiming to lose weight,
you may need to check your calorie
consumption. One typical technique is to cut
your daily consumption by 500–750
calories, which may help you lose roughly
1–2 pounds (0.5–1 kg) every week. That
being said, reducing your calorie intake too
much might be unproductive and damaging
to your health. Eating too few calories may
cause a drop in your metabolic rate or the
number of calories you burn daily.
Decreasing your calorie intake too much
may also produce a considerable drop in
lean body mass, which can limit the number
of calories that you burn at rest.

Furthermore, ingesting too few calories each day is related to various negative effects, including tiredness, headaches, nausea, dizziness, and irritability.

- **Eat extra fiber, particularly soluble fiber**

Eating soluble fiber may boost feelings of fullness, aid minimize the absorption of calories, and guard against the buildup of visceral fat around the organs. Soluble fibers absorb huge volumes of water and slow down the transit of food through the digestive system. This has been found to slow stomach emptying, allowing the stomach to enlarge and make you feel more full between meals.

Furthermore, soluble fiber may limit the number of calories your body can absorb from meals. Some study also shows that consuming more soluble fiber might be connected with less visceral fat, a form of fat that wraps around your organs — notably in the abdominal region — and is linked to various chronic health concerns. Good sources of soluble fiber include fruits, oats, barley, legumes, and some vegetables, such as broccoli and carrots.

- **Increase your consumption of probiotics**

Probiotics are a sort of helpful bacteria that may play a major function in weight control. Not only have some studies indicated that the gut microbiota may affect weight gain, but modifications in its makeup might also be connected to an increased risk of obesity. Regular use of probiotics may shift the balance toward good gut flora, lowering the risk of weight gain to help you attain and maintain a moderate weight. Some strains of probiotics have also been demonstrated to be especially helpful at helping decrease belly fat in those who are already living with obesity.

It's vital to realize that probiotics do not immediately induce weight reduction. They may be a valuable tool when taken in combination with a healthy diet and exercise, but they may not have the same impact on everyone. Always check with your doctor before choosing to add probiotics to your diet.

- **Add additional cardio to your program**

Doing cardio, or aerobic activity is a wonderful method to burn calories and enhance general health. Additionally, studies have shown that it's particularly efficient for strengthening your stomach and reducing belly fat. Studies normally suggest completing 150–300 minutes of moderate to high-intensity aerobic exercise weekly, which amounts to around 20–40 minutes each day. Examples of cardio include running, brisk walking, biking, and rowing.

- **Try protein shakes**

Protein smoothies are a simple way to add additional protein to your diet. Getting enough protein in your diet may temporarily enhance your metabolism, lessen your hunger, and help retain lean body mass.

Furthermore, studies show that increasing protein consumption may help decrease visceral fat, particularly if accompanied by a lower-calorie diet.
For optimum results, add additional nutrient-dense, fiber-rich items to your protein shake, such as spinach, kale, or berries.

- **Eat meals high in monounsaturated fatty acids**

Monounsaturated fatty acids are a kind of heart-healthy fat present in several meals. Interestingly, research reveals that diets rich in monounsaturated fatty acids may be connected with lower body weight. The Mediterranean diet is an example of a diet that's rich in monounsaturated fatty acids, and it's been linked to various health advantages, including a lower risk of weight gain and decreased belly fat in children and adults. Foods rich in monounsaturated fatty acids include olive oil, avocados, almonds, and seeds.

- **Limit your consumption of refined carbohydrates**

Limiting your carb consumption has been proved to provide actual health advantages, notably for weight reduction. More precisely, research demonstrates that low-carb diets may help decrease visceral fat and abdominal fat in certain individuals.

However, you don't have to take out all carbohydrates to gain the advantages, particularly if a low-carb diet is not optimal for your unique health history. Replacing refined carbohydrates, which are excessively processed and poor in critical nutrients like fiber, with whole grains may be extremely advantageous. Several studies have shown that eating more whole grains is associated with decreased body weight and belly fat.

- **Try resistance training**

Losing muscle mass is a typical adverse effect of dieting. This may lower your metabolic rate or the number of calories that you burn daily. Doing resistance workouts frequently may retain lean body mass and help you maintain or increase your metabolism. Moreover, resistance exercise may even be useful in reducing total body fat and visceral fat.

- **Do workouts standing instead of sitting**

If you're able, conducting workouts while standing up may enhance your health more than performing the same activities while sitting or using weight machines. By standing, you engage more muscles to maintain balance and hold up your weight. Therefore, you'll spend more energy working out.

Research comparing the effects of standing and sitting workouts indicated that certain standing activities enhanced muscular activation by 7–25%, compared to sitting. Another research revealed that standing may enhance your breathing and slightly boost your heart rate compared to sitting. Although this may seem like a little modification, for folks who can, standing might be a simple technique to strengthen the stomach and enhance your results.

- **Take walks regularly**

A mix of food and exercise is probably the most effective strategy to accomplish weight reduction and enhance your overall health.

Interestingly, studies have shown that you do not need to exercise intensely or spend hours at the gym to enjoy health advantages. Regular, brisk walks have been demonstrated to successfully decrease total body fat and the fat situated around the abdomen of persons currently living with obesity. One research indicated that when patients living with obesity completed 12,000 steps per day and conducted a brisk walk 3 days per week, they decreased visceral fat and hip circumferences after 8 weeks.

- **Limit sugary drinks**

Sugar-sweetened beverages including soda, fruit juice, sweet tea, and energy drinks are frequently rich in calories and added sugar. It's also quite simple to consume excessive volumes of these drinks at a time, which may considerably increase your daily calorie consumption and may lead to weight gain. This is because liquids have less of an impact on satiety compared to solid meals, making it simpler to eat them in excess. These beverages are also often rich with fructose, which has been linked directly to weight gain and increased belly fat.

- **Eat complete, single-ingredient meals**

Focusing on eating more complete, a single-ingredient meal is a wonderful strategy to boost the nutritional content of your diet. Whole foods are nutrient-dense and frequently high in fiber, which helps boost feelings of fullness to help you attain and maintain a healthy weight. Furthermore, several healthy whole foods have been demonstrated to promote weight control, including vegetables, nuts, and legumes.

- **Drink water**

There are various ways in which drinking more water might assist support weight control and reducing bloating. For starters, it may help weight reduction by very momentarily raising your metabolic rate or the number of calories that you burn at rest. Additionally, drinking water before meals might help you feel fuller, so you may consume fewer calories. What's more, boosting your water consumption may also help treat constipation, which can lead to bloating.

- **Practice mindful eating**

Mindful eating is a practice aimed to help you understand and manage your emotions and bodily feelings around food and hunger. It means slowing down, eating without distractions, concentrating on your body's hunger signals, and eating just until you feel full. Most studies agree that mindful eating helps enhance weight control by modifying your eating patterns and lowering stress-related behaviors, such as emotional eating or overeating. Also, it is more likely to help you sustain long-term weight reduction since it focuses on modifying your behavior and strengthening your relationship with food.

- **Limit carbonated beverages**

Drinking significant quantities of carbonated drinks such as soda or sparkling water might produce gas. This is because the bubbles in it contain carbon dioxide, which is produced from the liquid in your stomach. This may induce stomach distention or bloat. Chewing gum, sipping via a straw, or chatting while eating may all lead to bloating. Drinking from glass and changing fizzy beverages out for water may be good to help avoid bloating.

- **Try high-intensity interval training (HIIT)**

High-intensity interval training (HIIT) is a kind of exercise that generally includes completing periods of highly intense activity, such as sprinting, rowing, or jumping, with brief pauses in between. This technique of exercise helps your body burn more fat and temporarily raises your metabolic rate, even after you've done your workout. What's more, this sort of exercise takes up considerably less of your time than other types of exercise, since it normally can be accomplished in 10–20 minutes.

- **Manage your stress levels**

Not only has chronic stress been related to the development of various illnesses, but it also commonly leads to overeating and emotional eating, which may lead to weight gain. Additionally, stress leads the body to create cortisol, which is a hormone that has been found to boost hunger and food cravings.

Furthermore, some studies also show that increased accumulation of visceral fat might be connected to increased cortisol production as well, suggesting that stress may have a stronger impact on persons with more visceral fat. Though it may not be feasible to avoid stress altogether, adding stress-relieving activities to your daily routine, like yoga or meditation, might be useful.

- **Eat more protein**

Protein is a crucial component when it comes to weight reduction. High protein diets might lessen your appetite and promote feelings of fullness. Additionally, your body burns more calories digesting protein than fat or carbohydrates.

Protein may also assist keep lean body mass during weight reduction, which can help maintain your metabolism to facilitate weight control. How much protein you require depends on numerous variables, such as your age, sex, and activity level. For a simple approach to satisfy your protein requirements, make sure to include a solid source of protein — such as meat, fish, poultry, eggs, tofu, or lentils — in every meal.

• Track your food consumption

When you're attempting to lose weight, it might be useful to track your food consumption. There are various methods to accomplish this, but the most common and efficient alternatives include tracking calories or maintaining a food journal. You do not have to do this all the time, but it may be useful to keep track of your consumption for many days in a row every few weeks. This will make you more conscious of your calorie consumption and enable you to change your eating habits if required.

- **Add eggs to your diet**

Eggs are rich in protein and low in calories, with roughly 72 calories and 6 grams of protein in one large egg. Some study shows consuming eggs might aid with weight reduction. For example, one research found that participants who ate breakfast including eggs consumed fewer calories at lunch compared with those who ate a meal with cereal. Another research including over 2,200 people indicated that taking at least one egg per day was related to a 34% reduced risk of central obesity and a 38% lower risk of excess body fat. Similarly, research on over 24,000 participants indicated that eating eggs once a day was connected to a decreased incidence of abdominal obesity.

- **Get adequate sleep**

Getting a sufficient quantity of quality sleep each night is highly crucial for weight control. One research indicated that improved sleep health was connected with higher weight reduction and fat loss throughout a 12-month weight-loss intervention. Another small research in 36 persons revealed that obtaining 1 hour less of sleep for 5 nights per week was linked to slower fat reduction in those on a reduced calorie diet compared to a control group.

According to one research, sleep deprivation may be related to a greater risk of obesity, which might be owing to increased weariness and changes in levels of specific hormones that impact hunger and appetite. For most individuals, it's typically suggested to strive for at least 7 hours of sleep every night to promote overall health and keep a modest weight.

- **Try intermittent fasting**

Intermittent fasting is an eating pattern in which you alternate between eating and fasting for defined lengths of time. Two common intermittent fasting tactics include conducting a 24-hour fast two to four times per week or a 16/8 fast, where you limit your eating window to 8 hours each day, frequently by missing breakfast or having an early supper. Generally, this helps you consume fewer calories overall without having to deliberately think about it. While intermittent fasting has only been demonstrated to be as effective as regular, daily calorie restriction for reducing belly fat and promoting weight reduction, some people may find it easier to adhere to than other diets. Make careful to check with a doctor before starting intermittent fasting, since the long-term ramifications of this eating pattern are not yet understood.

- **Add fatty fish to your diet**

It's normally suggested to consume fatty fish once or twice every week. Fatty fish such as salmon, sardines, or tuna is a high-quality protein and rich in omega-3 acids. By consuming 2 to 3 pieces a week you may minimize the risk of ailments like heart disease and also burn your abdominal fat. Protein has been demonstrated to aid with weight reduction, and studies have revealed that omega-3 fatty acids may be connected to lower belly fat. While whole meals are typically the best method to acquire your vitamins and minerals, if you don't enjoy eating fatty fish, you can receive long-chain fatty acids from fish oil or fish oil supplements. Be cautious to check with a doctor first if you're contemplating supplementing.

- **Limit your consumption of added sugar**

Added sugar has been related to several chronic illnesses, including heart disease, type 2 diabetes, and fatty liver disease. It's recommended to limit added sugar intake to less than 10% of total daily calories. On a 2,000-calorie diet, this corresponds to around 200 calories, or 12 teaspoons (48 grams) each day. However, most people exceed this amount, and adults in the United States consume an average of 17 teaspoons (68 grams) of added sugar daily. Studies have shown a direct link between high intake of added sugar and increased waist size, especially in people who drink sugar-sweetened beverages. Added sugar is hidden in various foods, so it is very important to check the ingredient label carefully when shopping.

- ### **Replace some fat with MCT oil**

MCT oil is a type of oil that contains medium-chain triglycerides (MCTs). Studies suggest that replacing some dietary fat with MCT oil may increase energy expenditure and help you feel fuller. What's more, one review of 13 studies also found that MCTs were more effective at reducing body weight, total body fat, and belly fat compared with long-chain triglycerides. Keep in mind that MCT oil is still high in calories, much like other types of fat. Therefore, it's important not to just add MCT oil to your diet, but rather replace other sources of fat with it.

- ### **Strengthen your core**

Crunches and other abdominal exercises can help strengthen the muscles in your core. By doing regular core exercises, you can add mass to your abdominal muscles, which may improve your posture and enhance spinal stability to prevent injuries. Furthermore,

core exercises help you strengthen the muscles that ultimately hold in your belly, which may make you appear leaner.
If possible, aim to do core exercises that engage all your core muscles, such as planks or Pilates roll-ups.

- **Drink unsweetened coffee or green tea**

Unsweetened coffee and green tea are both very healthy liquids that may help you attain or maintain a modest weight. Several types of research have also indicated that consuming coffee and tea may be connected with lower belly fat and body weight. This may be partly owing to their caffeine content, which may temporarily enhance your metabolism to increase the number of calories that you burn throughout the day.

- **Limit alcohol intake**

Alcohol has seven calories for each gram, which partially explains why many alcoholic beverages are generally filled with liquid calories. Ounce for ounce, the beer carries a comparable number of calories as a sugary soft drink, but red wine contains almost double that much. Although moderate drinking is unlikely to alter body weight, excessive drinking is associated with greater weight gain, particularly around your midsection. According to the most current Dietary Guidelines for Americans, moderate drinking is defined as fewer than two drinks per day for males and less than one drink per day for women.

- **Sneak more activity into your day**

You may simply sneak more activity into your day by increasing the quantity of non-exercise activities you perform.

This entails walking, standing, fidgeting, or just generally moving about. According to one research, these activities may help you burn up to 2,000 more calories each day, depending on characteristics including your size and exercise level. Easy strategies to add additional exercise to your daily routine include walking about while chatting on the phone, standing up often, working at a standing desk, or using the stairs instead of the elevator whenever feasible.

The bottom line

If your doctor has recommended you to lose weight, or you have voluntarily taken the choice to drop some weight, it's crucial to keep your journey in perspective – no matter what random weight loss advertising and products attempt to tell you. It's not feasible to "target" fat reduction in only your stomach directly, but there are several ways that may assist promote total fat loss and weight loss efficiently.

In addition to making modifications to your food and training routine, getting enough sleep, regulating stress levels, and practicing mindful eating may all be useful. By adopting some of the suggestions described above into your daily routine, you may strive toward a "flatter stomach" while also improving your overall health.

Chapter 5

Lose Your Belly Fat By Exercising

As individuals become older, it's usual to observe an increase in belly fat gathering around the waistline. This is mainly because muscle mass declines with aging as fat accumulates. Belly fat might make you feel self-conscious or can create problems fitting into your favorite pair of clothes.

Exercises to Help Belly Fat

There are numerous workouts out there, but not all are made equal when it comes to eradicating belly fat. However, scientists and physicians alike agree that including physical exercise in your daily routine is a terrific strategy to burn off undesirable belly fat. Here are some workouts for belly fat that you may do to help you shrink down your waistline:

1. Aerobic or Cardio Exercise

Your first step in burning off visceral fat is integrating at least 30 minutes of aerobic activity or cardio into your daily regimen. Studies reveal that aerobic activities for belly fat assist to decrease belly fat and liver fat. Some fantastic cardio and aerobic activities for abdominal obesity include:

- Walking, particularly at a rapid speed

- Running

- Biking

- Rowing

- Swimming

- Cycling

- Group fitness courses

When picking a cardio exercise, make sure it's something that you love doing. This way, you're more motivated and will look forward to your training program.

2. HIIT or Interval Training

High-intensity interval training (HIIT) and interval training are fitness regimens that involve brief bursts of intensive activity mixed in with lower intensity motions and rest intervals. Research reveals that HIIT activities for belly fat assist to regulate weight and enhance your overall physical condition. These activities aren't overly time-consuming yet get your heart beating and train your whole body. Each program offers a range of exercises that incorporate the following movements:

- Pushing

- Pulling

- Squatting

- Deadlifting

3. Loaded carries

Typically, a HIIT regimen couples 30 seconds of hard exercise with 30 seconds of rest straight after before going on to the next activity. The procedure may be performed a few times to receive the best advantage. Some HIIT activities that individuals of all fitness levels and ages may attempt are:

- Jumping jacks

- Burpees

- Push-ups

- Jump squats

- High knees

To get started, pick a handful of HIIT workouts for belly fat. Perform one exercise for 30 seconds, then rest for 30 seconds. Do the next action, and then relax. When you complete all the activities, you may repeat the cycle a couple more times.

4. Abdominal Exercises

Because belly fat attaches to the waistline and stomach area, completing certain abdominal workouts might assist to battle it. They may assist to tone and flatten the stomach while giving you a fantastic source of exercise. These workouts are perfect for men and women of any age. Some abdominal workouts for belly fat that you may attempt at home include:

- 60-second planks

- Bicycle crunches

- Abdominal crunches

- Leg raises

5. Weight and Resistance Training

Weight training is also an essential component in burning off belly fat. Since muscles burn off more calories than fat does while the body is at rest, having a better muscular tone may allow you to burn off more fat. Researchers have also shown that resistance exercise, which includes weight training, may increase lean weight while lowering fat, and it can raise metabolism at the same time. Some weight training exercises for belly fat to incorporate into your regimen are:

- Bicep curls

- Lunges

- Squats

- Tricep kick-backs

With these exercises, you may complete 12 repetitions with lesser weights, between five and eight pounds. Another alternative is to utilize heavier weights with fewer repetitions and rest time between sets.

Safety Considerations

While it's necessary to obtain at least 30 minutes of moderate exercise a day, you don't want to overtrain and push yourself too hard. Sometimes when you overtrain, your body might create too much cortisol. This is a stress hormone that is related to belly fat, thus overtraining may make it more difficult to burn off belly fat. Just keep in mind the suggestions for moderate frequent activity, and consult with your doctor if you have concerns about how else your exercise regimen might improve your waistline.

Chapter 6

Belly Friendly Recipes

While spot-reducing belly fat is not exactly possible, eating fewer calories than you burn translates to overall weight loss—including your belly. Eating for weight loss is very specific and requires a few essential components.

Essential Tips For Belly Fat Loss

Protein: Important for feeling full, preserving muscle mass, and improving our metabolism, protein is key at each meal while trying to lose weight.

Fiber: High-fiber carbs, vegetables, and fruits are invaluable during a weight loss diet to feel both full and satisfied. Focusing on about a cup of carbs at each meal is a good place to start for most.

Volume: When you have to eat a little less, it's helpful to add more to your plate to feel less deprived. Fruits and veggies are a great "add" to the diet to increase the total volume of food without extreme restrictions. Focus on half your plate coming from veggies at one main meal to get started.

A calorie-conscious mindset: You don't have to start counting every calorie to lose weight. However, it helps to be conscious of the high-calorie foods in your diet, and begin making swaps. Trade out the creamy dressings for lighter sauces, switch high-fat meats for leaner cuts and swap dessert for a lighter option.

If you're one of those people who tend to carry weight in their belly, you can do something about it! While hundreds of crunches aren't exactly the answer, what you put in your mouth is. Certain foods are proven to diminish belly fat, like whole grains, MUFAs like avocado, nuts, seeds, and olive oil.

You can also eat eggs, lean protein (especially fish like salmon), and tofu. Fiber-rich veggies such as greens and beans fight visceral fat around your inner organs, as well as berries like blueberries and raspberries. This is great news! Make one of these delicious dinner recipes tonight, and with each bite, you can feel good that you're doing your body and your belly good.

Below are some delicious and weight loss-friendly meals that can be incorporated into your daily meal plan.

- Black Bean Omelet

- Grilled Pork Tenderloin with salad

- Grilled Mahi-Mahi with Salsa Verde

- Healthier Grilled Caesar Salad

- Hearty Turkey Chili

- Moroccan-Inspired Quinoa Pilaf and Salmon

- Baked Chicken with Tomatoes and Capers

- Teriyaki Pork Chops with Sauteed Apples

- Easy Chicken Tortilla Soup

- Chicken Cacciatore

- Chicken Mole Enchiladas

- Healthy Chicken Tikka Masala

- Greek Salad Recipe with Chicken

- Spanish Garlic Shrimp

- Pumpkin Mole Chili

- Paleo Turkey Bolognese with Garlic Spaghetti Squash

- Butternut Squash Hash

- Instant Pot Chicken and Rice Soup

- Overnight Chia Pudding

- Minestrone Soup with Pesto

- Breakfast Hash with Sweet Potato and Chicken Sausage

- Spicy-Sweet Grilled Chicken Pineapple Sandwich

www.ingramcontent.com/pod-product-compliance
Lightning Source LLC
Chambersburg PA
CBHW051449150726

48000CB00005B/2318